Belabbas Rafik

Physiology of rabbit reproduction

Belabbas Rafik

Physiology of rabbit reproduction

educational book

ScienciaScripts

Imprint

Any brand names and product names mentioned in this book are subject to trademark, brand or patent protection and are trademarks or registered trademarks of their respective holders. The use of brand names, product names, common names, trade names, product descriptions etc. even without a particular marking in this work is in no way to be construed to mean that such names may be regarded as unrestricted in respect of trademark and brand protection legislation and could thus be used by anyone.

Cover image: www.ingimage.com

This book is a translation from the original published under ISBN 978-620-6-70157-6.

Publisher:
Sciencia Scripts
is a trademark of
Dodo Books Indian Ocean Ltd. and OmniScriptum S.R.L publishing group

120 High Road, East Finchley, London, N2 9ED, United Kingdom
Str. Armeneasca 28/1, office 1, Chisinau MD-2012, Republic of Moldova, Europe
Printed at: see last page
ISBN: 978-620-7-78983-2

Contents

CHAPTER I

Introduction

The domestic rabbit (*Oryctolagus cuniculus*) is both a laboratory animal and a production animal (meat, fur or hair). The rabbit is highly prolific, with short gestation and lactation periods and a production rate of up to 61 kg per female rabbit per year. It has a rapid growth rate and a highly nutritious meat (low in fat and cholesterol but rich in proteins). All these characteristics make the rabbit a very interesting zootechnical species.

Reproduction in rabbits is a key stage in the creation of new breeds, the transmission of genetic progress and, above all, the success of breeding. The way in which rabbits are bred has changed considerably, particularly since the early 1990s when artificial insemination began to be used by breeders, especially in Europe. Artificial insemination has helped to change the way breeding is organised on farms, insofar as it has led to the development of single-batchery breeding.

In order to facilitate the application of biotechnologies (artificial insemination, oestrus synchronisation and embryo transfer) and the improvement of reproductive performance by genetic means, a minimum knowledge of rabbit reproductive physiology is required.

This book looks at the anatomical, physiological and zootechnical features of reproduction in the rabbit.

I. The female genital tract :

I.1 Anatomy of the female genital tract :

The organisation of the female дёпка1 apparatus is identical to that of other mammals. This apparatus brings together (**Figure 1,2,3**):

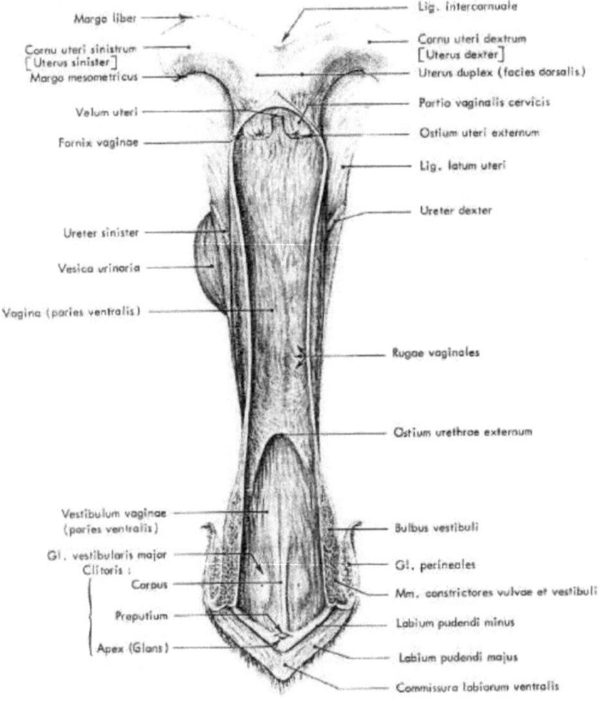

Figure 1: The дёпH^ apparatus of the rabbit.

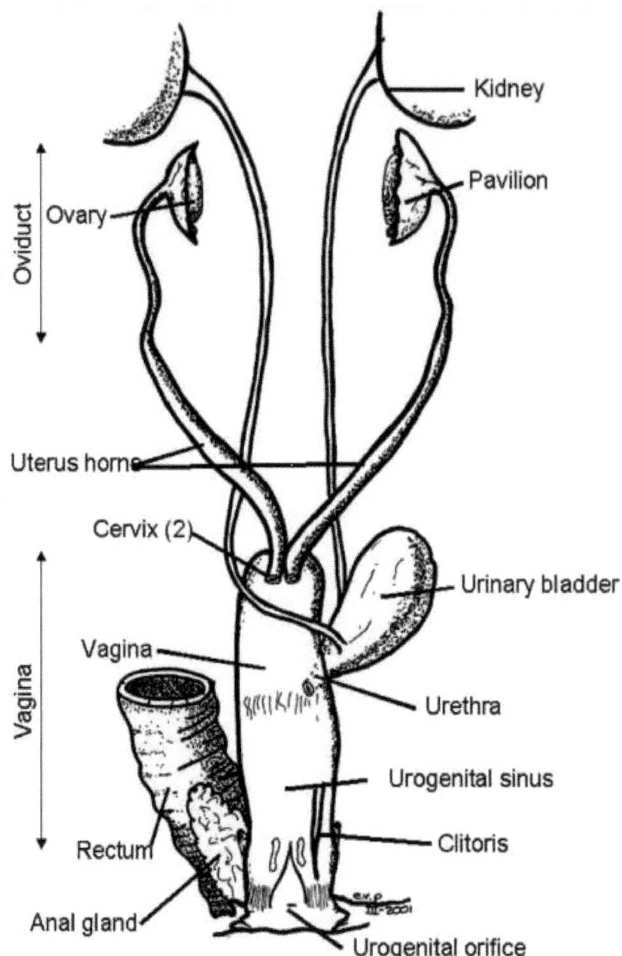

Figure 2: Schematic presentation of the female genital tract.

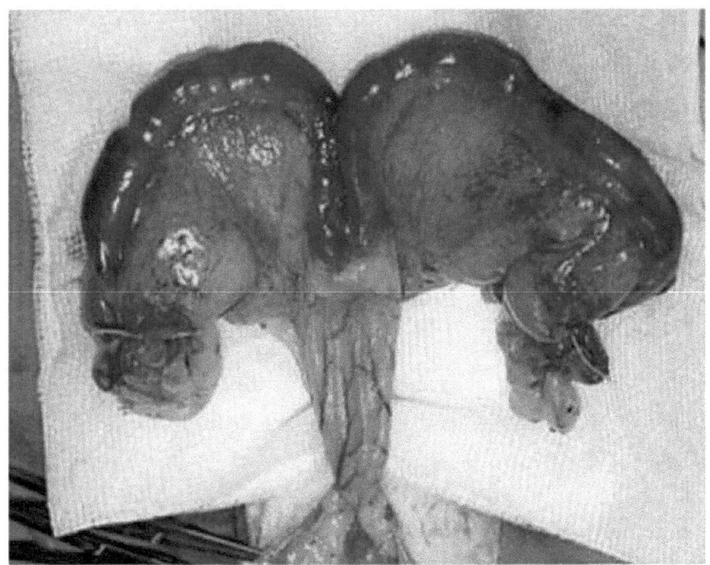

Figure 3: Photo of 1 female дёпка1 device.

- **Ovaries :**

The ovaries, of which there are two, are ovoid and reach 1 to 2 cm at their largest (**Figure 4**). They are where the female gametes are prepared.

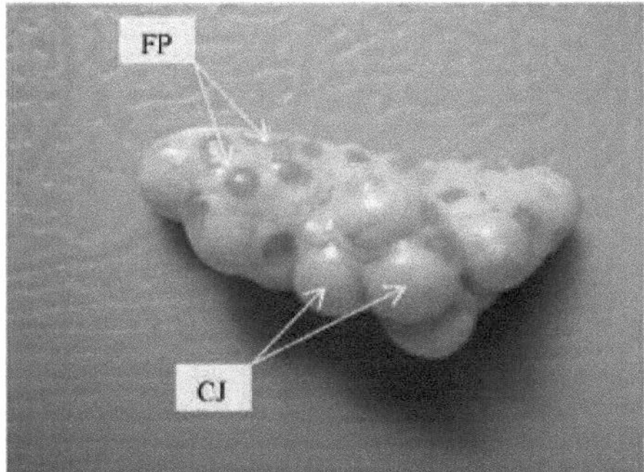

Figure 4: Ovary of a pregnant rabbit (**FP:** Preovulatory follicles; **CJ**: Yellow bodies).

- **Oviducts :**

These are small ducts 10 to 16 cm long, composed of the pavilion, ampulla and isthmus and 1oca1isës under each ovary.

> *The Pavilion* is calyx-shaped, very dëve1oppë, and collects the ovule at the time of egg-laying.

> *The ampulla* is the site of fëcondation. The 1umiëre of this tube contains numerous

5

^Hёcв cells allowing the gamëtes to be transported.

> ***The isthmus*** is a much narrower duct lined with mucus and sëcrëtrice cells but with far fewer ciliated cells. It opens into the uterine horn at the level of the utero-tubal junction.

- The uterus :

Although externally the uterine horns are united in their posterior part into a single body, in reality there are two indëpendent uteruses of around 7 cm, opening sëparëmentally via two cervical ducts into the vagina, which is 6 to 10 cm long. The whole is supported by the broad ligament which has four main points of attachment under the vertebral column.

1.2. The development of the gonads :

After birth, the ovaries develop much more slowly than the rest of the body. An acceleration is observed from 50 to 60 days (**Figure 5**). Primordial follicles appear from 13eme days after birth and the first antrum follicles around 65 to 70 days.

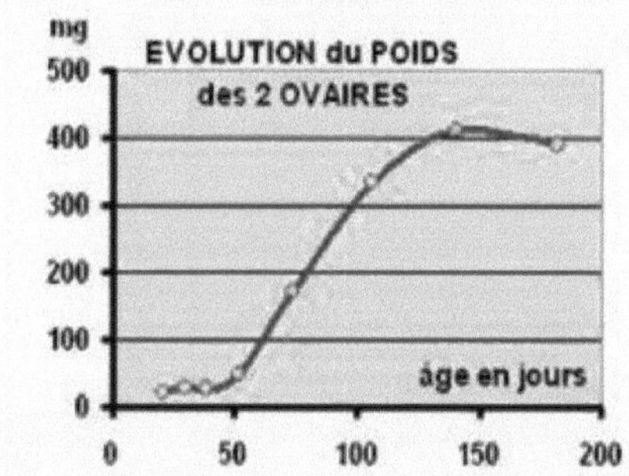

Figure 5: Changes in the weight of the two ovaries.

1.3. Sexing :

Sexing is an essential step in separating young of different sexes or in forming pairs at the time of breeding. In the male, a short penis pointing backwards can be seen, while in the female, a fairly prominent vulva can mimic a small penis, but it is split, whereas the opening of the male's sheath is circular (**Figure 6**).

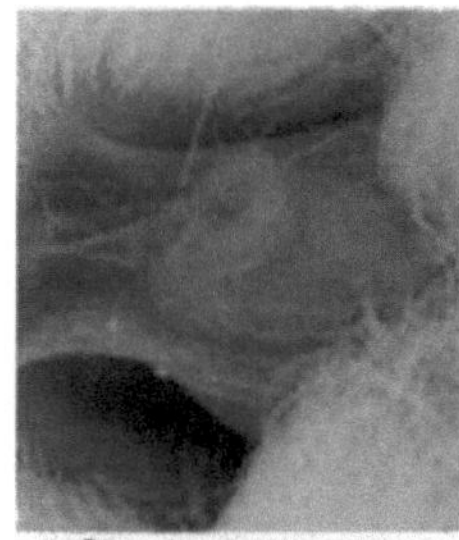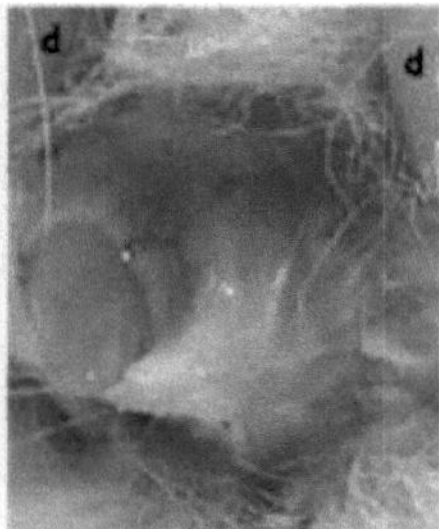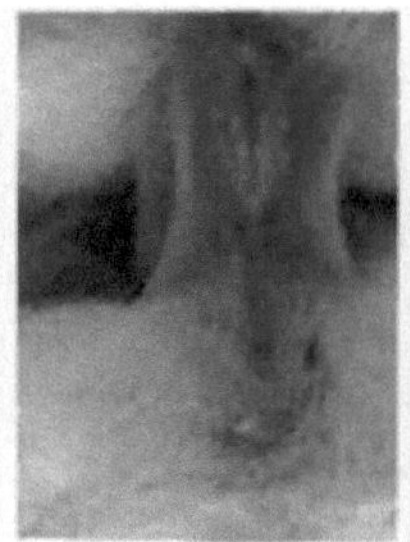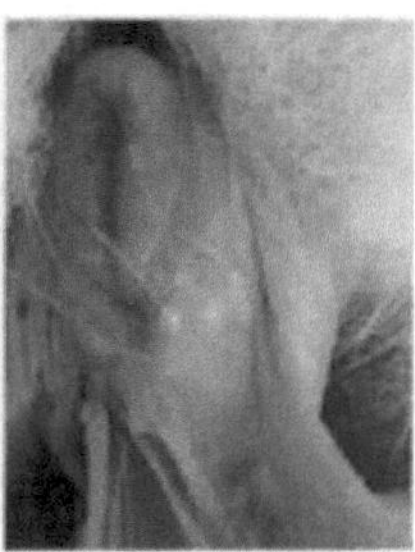

Figure 6: Sexing in rabbits.

II. Sexual activity in rabbits :

II.1. Puberty and age at first bleeding :

II.1.1. Puberty :

Puberty must be considered in its дёгёпёral sense, including all the morphological, physiological and behavioural changes that occur in the growing individual. In the rabbit, puberty is reached around the age of 3 to 7 months. The age of puberty, i.e. the age at which mating leads to ovulation for the first time, is poorly defined and depends on a number of factors:

• **Breed**: Precocity appears to be better in small and medium-sized breeds (4 to 6 months) than in large breeds (5 to 8 months).

• **Body development** : The more rapid the growth, the greater the precocity. Most females are pubëres as soon as they reach 75% of their adult weight, but it is prëfërable to wait until they have reached 80% of this weight.

• **Diet** : Dietary restriction or poor diet during the përiode of growth will delay puberty.

• **Photoperiod**: Females born in autumn and which consequently reach puberty in spring are earlier than females born in spring. Also, exposure to prolonged ëclairement favours the onset of puberty and amplifies restral behaviour.

II.1.2. Age at first mating :

The first mating should take place when the animal presents a physical conformation and a sexual maturity corresponding to the breed to which it belongs. However, this mating is often anticipated, in order to exploit the animal more advantageously and also to prevent it from fattening excessively. Many breeders and spëcialists prefer to base their judgement of aptitude for reproduction on the animal's weight rather than its age. The weight must represent more than 80% of the optimal weight for an adult. However, the age at sexual maturity varies from breed to breed, with giant breeds often maturing later. The first male acceptances can take place as early as 13 to 14 weeks of age in medium breeds, but it is advisable to avoid breeding animals that are too young or insufficiently developed (not before 16-17 weeks).

II.2. l/restriis and the oestrien cycle :

The estrous cycle is the time interval between 2 consëcutifs restrus in female cycles. It is specific to each species (21 days in cows, 17 to 18 days in ewes). The rabbit, on the other hand, does not have an estrous cycle with regular heats during which ovulation occurs spontaneously. They are considered to be in more or less permanent oestrus, and only ovulate if there is a coi't. This is known as induced ovulation. The duration of oestrus or dioestrus varies from one rabbit to another; some may be in effective oestrus for 28 consecutive days, while others may be in oestrus for only 2 days in 4 weeks (**Figure 7**).

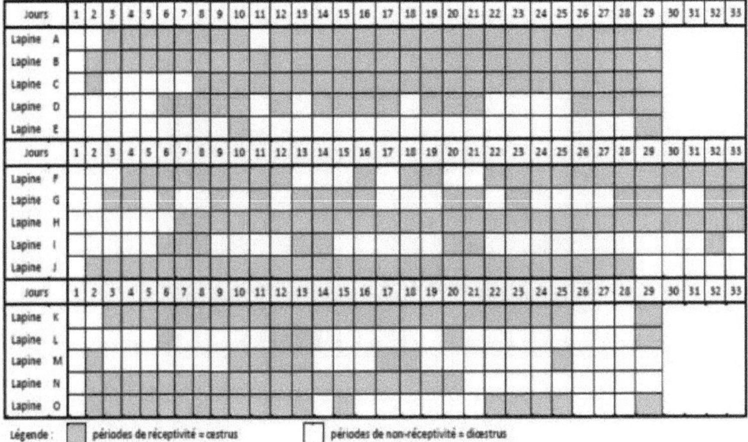

Figure 7: Rëceptivitë and acceptance of male in nulliparous pubëer rabbits.

11.2.1. The components of sexual behaviour :

In female mammifëres, we can distinguish three components of sexual behaviour:

- *The attraction phase*: I . Attractivity is the set of signals that orientate the male towards the female or, more simply, is defined as the attraction of the male to the female (**Figure 8**). Pheromones acting as sexual attractants have been identified.

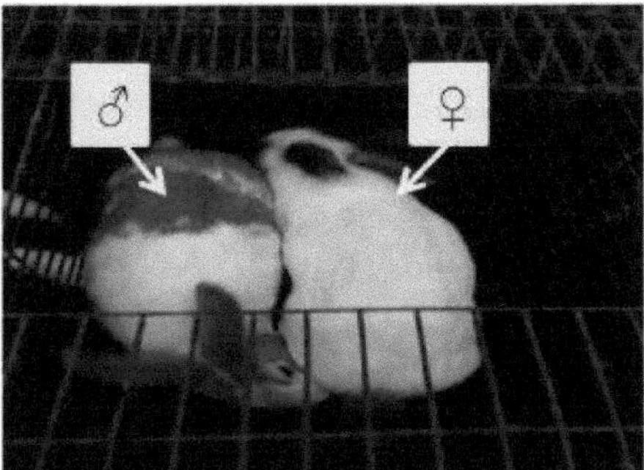

Figure 8: The attraction phase.

- *The precopulatory phase*: This corresponds to proceptivity in the female. It describes the female's active search for the male. It includes all the behaviours aimed at the male and which have the effect of establishing or maintaining sexual interaction (**Figure 9**). The female rabbit marks different objects with chin secretions. The male and female try to sniff each other and chase each other by turning rapidly. Proceptivity is also marked by an increase in the female's motor activity. The female rabbit circles the male, lifting and wagging her tail laterally (**Figure 9**).

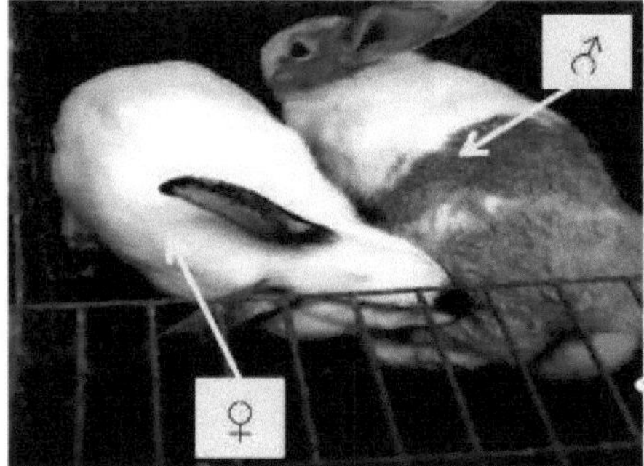

Figure 9: The precopulatory phase.

• **_Receptivity_**: this is the main indicator of oestrus. It qualifies the state of the female that accepts mating. At the moment of overlap, the male makes pelvic movements that stimulate the female. The female quickly adopts a particular position, called lordosis, characterised by the convex curvature of her bitter train (**Figure 10**).

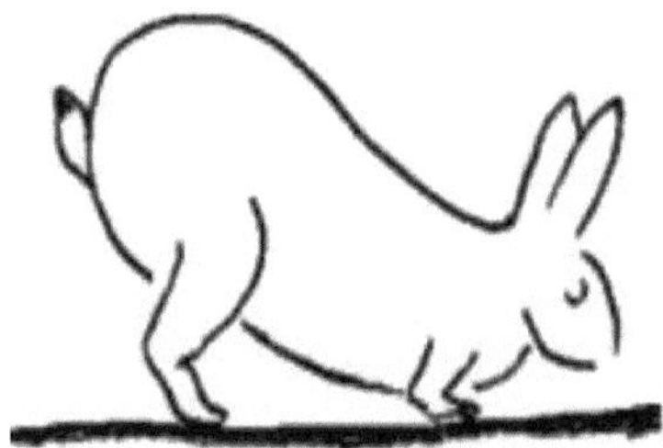

Figure 10: The lordosis position.

The female rests on her belly, raising her hindquarters slightly to make it easier for her to move.

intromission (**Figure 11**).

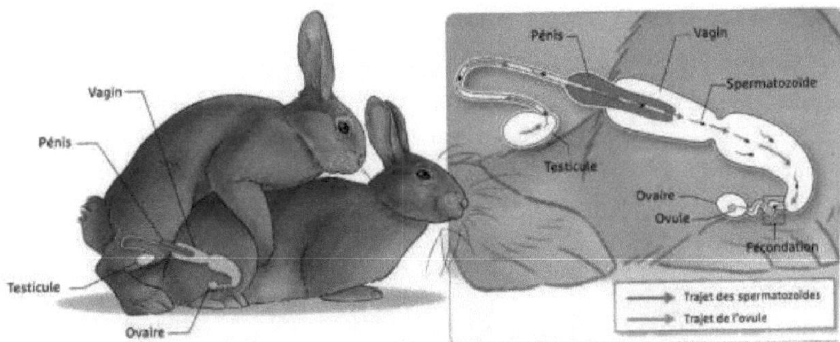

Figure 11: Mating in rabbits.

The lordosis position is an innate motor reflex inherited by the hypothalamus. However, during oestrus, the restrogenes break this inhibition and as soon as the male mounts the female, tactile stimuli on the flanks and rump trigger reflex contraction of the muscles, causing curvature of the vertebral column (**Figure 12**).

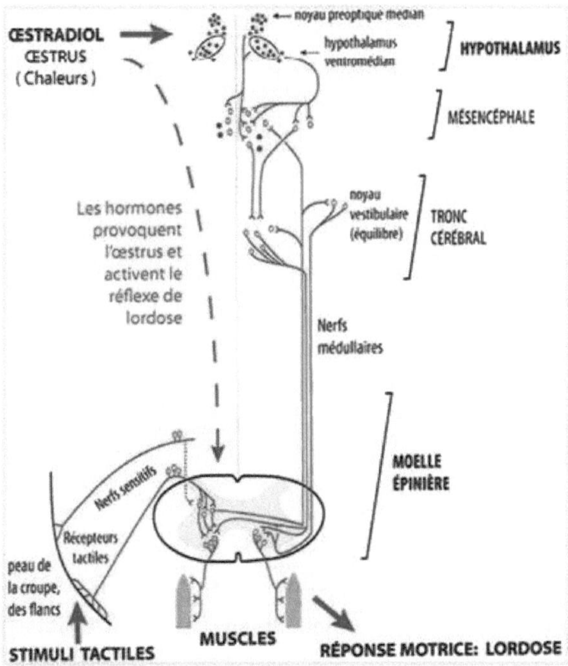

Figure 12: Neural organisation of lordosis.

On the other hand, if the female rabbit is in direstrus or not receptive, she will refuse to mate and will huddle in a corner of the cage or become aggressive towards the male.

11.2.2. Morphological changes associated with oestrus :

Receptivity is Hëc to morphological changes in the vulva. Four colours of vulva, linked or not to a state of turgidity, have been described in rabbits: white, pink, red and violet (**Figure 13**). Male acceptance was highest when the vulva was red and turgid, and lowest when the vulva was white and non-turgid. In addition, vulval turgidity significantly increased the receptivity rate for all vulval colours.

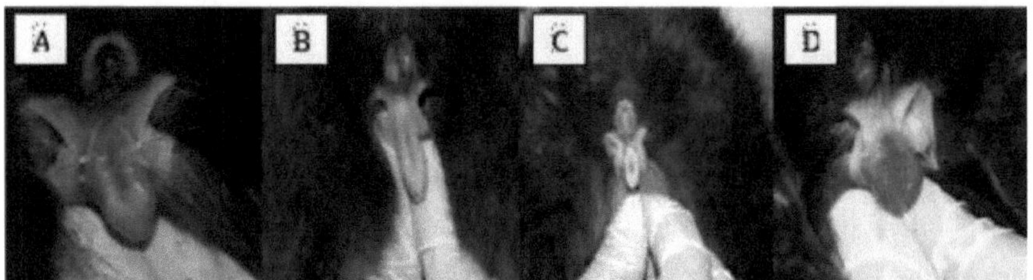

Figure 13 : Aspects of the vulva in the female rabbit. **A**: turgid pink; **B**: turgid white;

C: white, non-turgid; **D**: red, turgid

During oestrus, large quantities of restrogen are secreted, causing hyperhemia of the vulval lips and intensifying the colour and tumefaction of the vulva. Injecting restrogen into an ovariectomised rabbit increases blood flow to the genital tract. Restrogen induces vasodilation by relaxing the smooth muscle fibres of the blood vessels (by binding to their membrane receptors). Under the action of restrogens, endothelial cells release nitric oxide or nitric monoxide, which relaxes smooth muscle fibres.

11.2.3. Control of frestrus in rabbits :

Restrus is related to the ëvolutive stage of foLLIculogënëse. The cells of the internal theca surrounding each preovulatory follicle, sëcrete restrogens in proportion to their mass. The circulating level of these hormones is therefore only ëĸyë when a sufficient number of mature follicles are present on the ovary. Also, bi^ral oophorectomy abolishes sexual behaviour in rabbits.

11.2.3.1.   Ovarian control of oestris :

- Folliculogenesis from conception to puberty (Figure 14):

On day 16ème of embryonic development, sexual differentiation is established. Unlike most mammals (ewes, cows,...), the stock of primordial follicles in the rabbit is not depleted during foetal life but becomes established during the ^onatal përiod (first few weeks after birth). The rabbit is born with immature gonads containing only oogonia. These cells multiply with intense mitotic activity between 16eme and 18eme days *post cottum*.

From the first day after birth, the entry into prophase of the first mëiotic division corresponds to the diffèrenciation of the ovogonia into oocytes at the germinal vësicle (GV) stage.

___

__At 14eme days after birth__, the stock of oocytes is defined. At this point, the size of the follicular reserve has been determined and will diminish progressively during the animal's life (atresia or ovulation).

__By 20eme days after birth__, all oocytes are blocked at the diplotëne stage of prophase I and are predominantly in the form of primordial follicles. The signals that induce the growth of quiescent primordial follicles are still poorly understood and result in the formation of primordial follicles with a layer of ovoid peripheral follicular cells. Follicular growth then continues progressively until formation of the antral cavity or antrum, which appears, as in most other mammals, when the follicle has reached a diameter of approximately 200 pm. The first secondary, tertiary and antrum follicles appear at 4, 8 and 12 weeks after birth respectively. At this stage, the appearance of the first antrum follicles does not mark the establishment of puberty in the rabbit because the immaturity of the ovarian structures and hormonal system does not allow these follicles to develop to the pre-ovulatory stage.

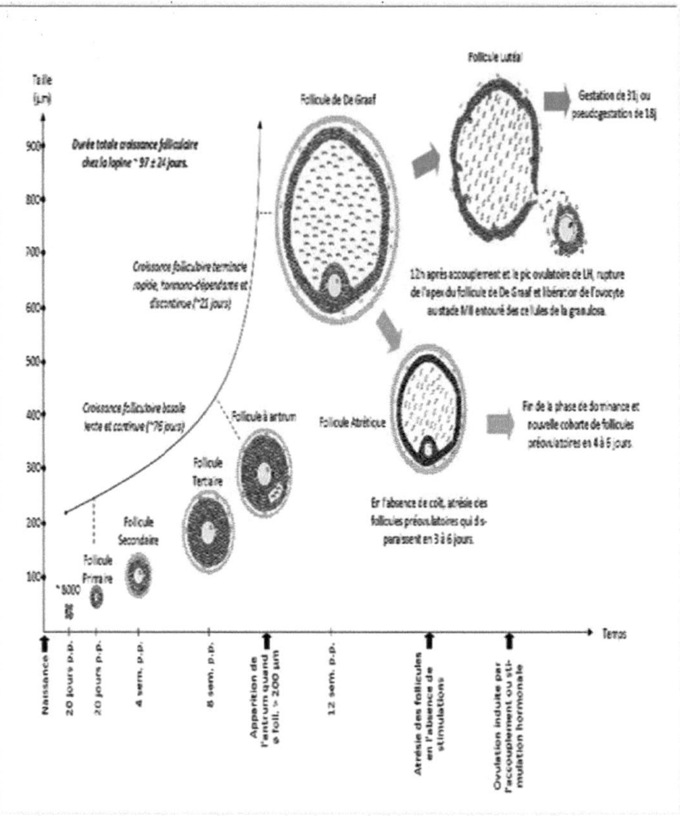

Figure 14: Schematic diagram of folliculogenesis in the rabbit.

"Folliculogenesis in the pubescent female:

The rabbit is a non cyclë animal that produces continuously mature follicles that become atretic if ovulation is not induced. Histological ëtudes rëalisëes in the rabbit have shown the existence of 5 types of follicles in the absence of mating (**Table 1**) :

Table 1: The different classes of ovarian follicle.

Types of follicle	Histological characteristics
Primordial follicle	Formed by a layer of flattened follicle cells, with less than ten cells surrounding an oocyte I blocked in the prophase of the 1er meiotic division.
Primary follicle	Has a single layer of follicular cells in a cubic shape called the granulosa

Secondary follicle	There are two to four layers of cubic cells around the oocyte and at this stage the zona pellucida appears.
Tertiary or antral follicle (cavitary).	Formation of four to five layers of follicular cells and appearance of a small antral cavity.
The large antral follicle known as the De Graaf follicle	It has more than five layers of granulosa cells and contains a large cavity or antrum. The oocyte is pushed towards the periphery and the granulosa is organised into the membrana granulosa resting on Slavjanski's basal lamina and the corona radiata and cumulus oophorus around oocyte II.

In the pubertal rabbit, there are two phases in follicle development. Basal follicular growth (independent of gonadotropic secretions) and terminal follicular development, which is dependent on gonadotropins, including FSH, which promotes the multiplication of granulosa cells and therefore follicle growth.

As soon as the antrum appears, the mature oocyte I enters its maturation phase and becomes oocyte II. The number of mature follicles is relatively constant between individuals with, at any one time, 8 follicles likely to develop until ovulation. In the absence of stimulation, the mature follicles present on the surface of the ovary have a lifespan of 7 to 10 days or 3 to 6 days, before regressing by atresia. Following follicular dëgënëration, the rate of restrogënes decreases and the rabbit is no longer receptive. The "dioestrus" phase therefore corresponds to the phase of dëgënëration of the follicles. In theory, it lasts 1 to 4 days.

### 11.2.3.2.	Hormonal control of oestrus :

Several hormones are involved in controlling oestrus in the rabbit:

Wstrogens: term used to describe any substance with hormonal activity that stimulates the development and function of the female organs. Restrogënes are necessary for sexual receptivity in the rabbit and immunisation against 17-в restradiol prevents oestrus. They are secreted by the ovaries (17-B-restradiol and restrone) but also by the placenta during gestation (restriol). In the ovary, restrogens are secreted by the cells of the inner lip of the follicles. Their circulating level therefore depends on follicular development. In ovariectomised rabbits, administration of restradiol benzoate restores lordosis, showing behaviour and marking by the chin glands. These behaviours result from the action of restrogen on the ventro-lateral zone of the hypothalamus.

Progesterone: After ovulation, its release by the ovaries into the bloodstream is enabled by follicle revolution in particular by the penetration of blood vessels between the granulosa cells during the formation of corpora lutea. From mid-gestation, progesterone is also sëcrëtëed by the placenta. In rabbits, progestërone inhibits follicular growth and stëroidogëne activity of the ovary. Contrary to what has been ële dëcribed in rats and mice, in rabbits progërone has no stimulatory effect on sexual behaviour and its blood level is very low during oestrus. Injection of progestërone to an ovariectomisedëe rabbit inhibits lordosis and marking by the mentoniëres glands.

Androgens: **A** family of stëroid hormones with a masculinising effect. In rabbits, they are synthëtisëed by the internal theca of the ovarian follicles, the interstitial glands of the ovary and the suprarenals. In the ovariectomisëe rabbit, androgenes cause the appearance of oestrus behaviour. Also, active immunisation against testostërone inhibits the onset of sexual receptivity. The effect of androgens on sexual receptivity results from their aromatisation into restrogens.

III. Reproduction and ovulation:

III.1.   1. Breeding:

Mating takes place in the male's cage, not the other way round: otherwise, she can be very aggressive in her territory and cause him serious injury. Outside his territory, the male will tend to spend his time marking everything around him instead of looking after the female. If the female is receptive and the male is sexually active, the mating time is around 10 to 20 seconds. The female stops when the male tries to mount her and adopts the lordosis position. Mating is very rapid, accompanied by a cry from the male, who quickly withdraws and throws himself to the side after ejaculation (**Figure 15**).

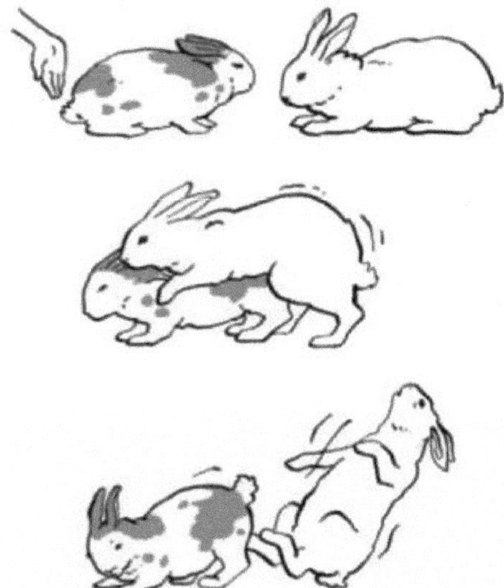

Figure 15: Mating in rabbits.

The frequency of use of the male influences the volume, motility, concentration and viability of the sperm. When the male is used at a rate of one service every day, the volume of ejaculate decreases from 0.79 to 0.54 ml, its concentration decreases from 286.14 x 10^6 to 231.66 x 106/ml and the percentage of live spermatozoa from 78.6% to 73.2% compared with use at a rate of one service every 3 days. Several authors point out that, in principle, each breeder should only service three females a week, with a one-day rest period after each service.

III.2.   2. Ovulation :

In species with spontaneous ovulation, an increasing increase in restrogens past a threshold concentration exerts a positive feedback control on the hypothalamus, inducing ovulation via the hypothalamic-pituitary-gonadal axis. In contrast, in the rabbit, a species with induced ovulation, there is no such feedback. Restrogen production only affects the rabbit's sexual behaviour. In the rabbit, ovulation is a neuroendocrine reflex induced by stimuli associated with mating or by the use of exogenous hormones. Ovulation can also be triggered by mechanical stimulation, overlap between females or with a sterilised male. Ovulation involves two different pathways: the afferent pathway, which transmits the stimuli associated with coi't to the central nervous system via the nerves, and the efferent pathway which, via the humoral pathway, allows oocyte maturation (nuclear maturation) to be completed and ovulation to occur (**Figure 16**).

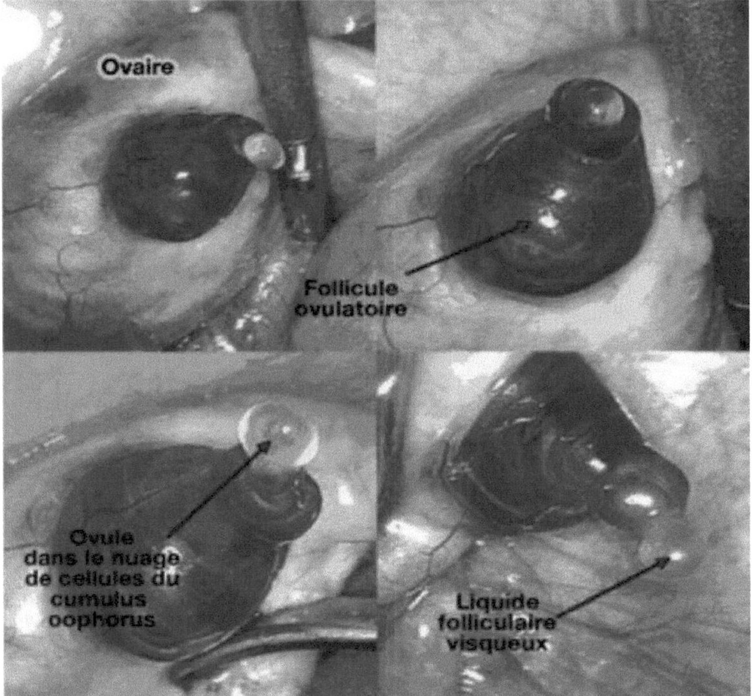

Figure 16: Mechanism of ovulation and follicular rupture.

- **The related track :**

Mating causes stimuli to be sent in the form of 2 pieces of information via different nerve pathways:

> Erotic messages, probably reflecting the quality of the court.

> Information specific to the coupling.

The resulting nerve impulse is transmitted to the brain and then to the rhinencephalon, which also integrates other types of internal (stëroid concentration, for example) and external (olfactory, pheromone, gustatory, visual, auditory) messages. Finally, the order is transmitted to the hypothalamus, which converts the electrical messages into hormonal messages.

- **The efferent path :**

Sensory impulses, induced by copulation-vaginal and cervical stimulation-are delivered via an ascending nerve pathway to the hypothalamus, where they trigger a release of GnRH that occurs 20 to 40 minutes after mating (**Figure 17**). The neurotransmitters involved are noradrenaline and acetylcholine.

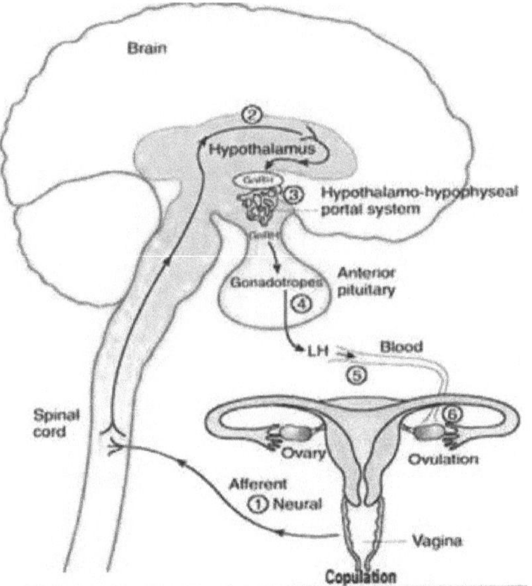

Figure 17: The neuroendocrine ovulation reflex.

GnRH reaches the pituitary almost immediately via the hypothalamic-pituitary portal system (low concentration in the blood to avoid dilution of the hormone) (**Figure 18**). This molecule is secreted in regular, low-amplitude pulses during oestrus. However, during mating, GnRH discharge increases 40-fold.

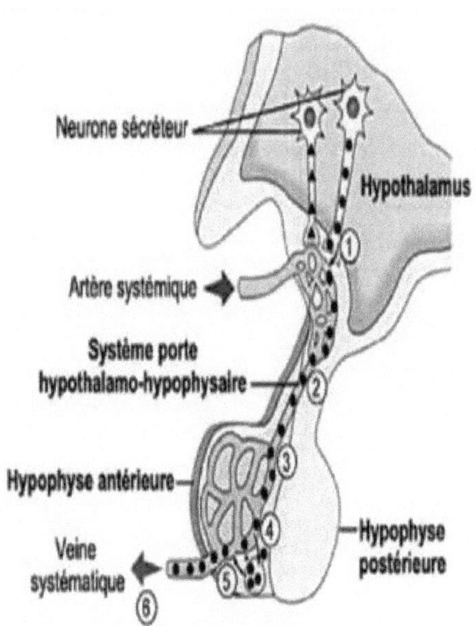

Figure 18: The hypothalamic-pituitary portal system.

GnRH acts on the anterior pituitary gland, which in turn releases 2 gonadotropins:

> *LH*: a glycopeptide molecule made up of around 200 amino acids. Its peak

is observed around 2 hours after coi't, then becomes low after 12 hours.

It allows the maturation of the large antrum follicles and triggers ovulatory egg-laying approximately 10 to 12 hours after coi't. Following ovulation, a scar called the "stigma" corresponding to the rupture of the përiphëric layers and the inflammatory reactions associated with ovulation remains visible on the apical part of the ovulating follicles (**Figure 19**). The number of ova produced by the left and right ovaries is comparable during the same ovulation. In addition, LH is responsible for the elevation of blood progestagens.

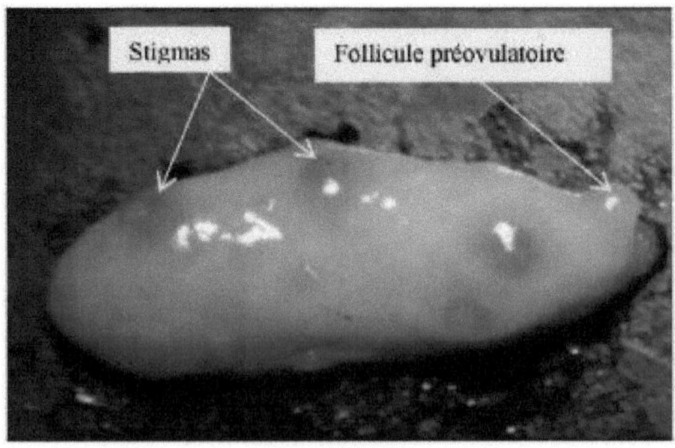

Figure 19: The stigmas or ovulation points on an ovary of a female rabbit.

> *FSH*: a glycopeptide molecule made up of around 200 amino acids. Post-coital development is biphasic, with the 1er peak synchronous with LH and the 2eme peak around 24 to 48 hours after coitus (**Figure 20**). The role of FSH in the rabbit is essentially to trigger the resumption of meiosis up to metaphase II. The 2eme FSH peak is responsible for the recruitment and development of growing follicles and stimulates the synthesis of restrogens (which have a luteotrophic action in the rabbit and maintain the activity of the corpora lutea).

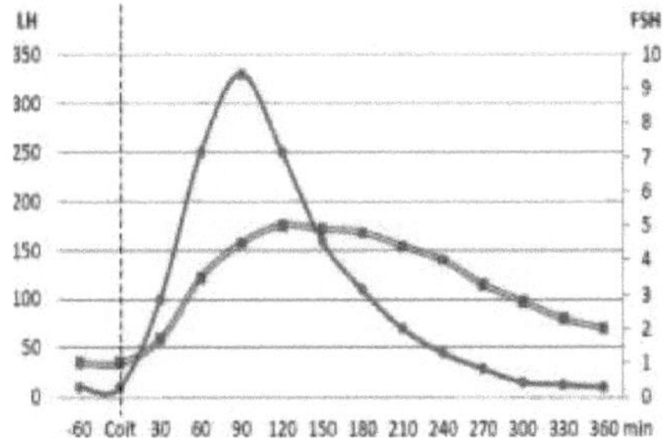

Figure 20: post coi't plasma LH and FSH levels.

Furthermore, in the minute following mating, oxytocin levels increase while prolactin levels decrease (**Figure 21**). A double oxytocin discharge is observed. The 1ere discharge is synchronous with that of LH and FSH, the 2eme occurs 5 hours after coitus. The function of this oxytocin discharge appears to be to allow spermatozoa to cross the uterine cervix and begin to progress into the uterus. Mating also induces a rapid and significant release of prolactin. This is concomitant with the release of LH. It helps to maintain a progesterone state favourable to implantation by stimulating steroidogenesis by the corpora lutea.

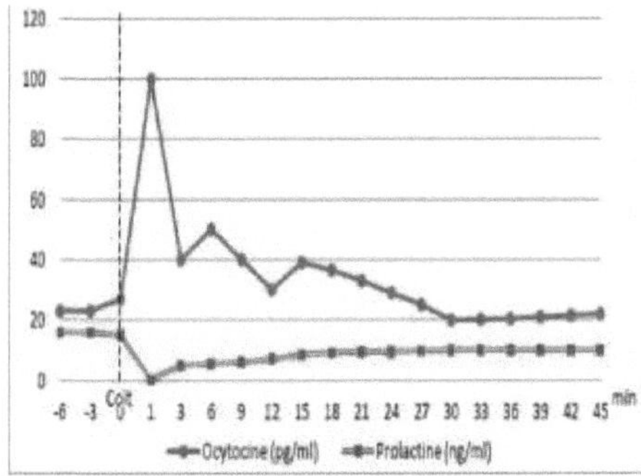

Figure 21: Post-coital plasma levels of oxytocin and prolactin.

Recent studies on llamas and alpacas have shown that ovulation is induced not only by mating but also by a factor present in seminal plasma. In fact, injection of 2 ml of seminal plasma intramuscularly in these animals caused a peak in plasma LH 75 minutes after treatment and resulted in ovulation in over 90% of cases.

IV. Post-ovulatory physiology :

IV.1. Sperm upwelling :

As soon as they are released, the oocytes are "aspirated" by the pinnae of the oviduct and can be fecundated, with a maximum fecundity between 12 and 15 *hpost coitum (p.c.)* before gradually decreasing until 19 hp.c. when the oocytes begin to degenerate. The spermatozoa deposited in the upper part of the vagina pass through the cervix autonomously. Muscular movements of the vagina can also help sperm to pass through the cervix. Of the 150 to 200 million spermatozoa ejaculated, only 2 million (1%) will be present in the uterus, encountering obstacles mainly on their way up to the uterine cervix and the utero-tubal junction.

The time taken for the spermatozoids to reach the distal part of the ampulla varies according to the authors, ranging from 30 minutes after coitus to 8 hours *p.c.* In the uterus, the spermatozoa come into contact with uterine secretions, which form a liquid medium favourable to their progress. This is ensured by muscular contractions of the uterus. The level of hormones circulating in the rabbit has a direct influence on the success of fertilisation. Restrogen encourages sperm to ascend into the uterus, while progesterone inhibits their passage to the cervix. Prostaglandins are also involved in promoting muscular contractions in the uterus. A release of oxytocin allows the spermatozoa to pass through the cervix and begin to progress into the uterus.

IV.2 Capacity building :

The spermatozoon coming from the tail of the epididymis or ejaculate can only express its fecundity after a stay of several hours in the female's genital tract. The changes that the spermatozoon must undergo to acquire the ability to fertilise an oocyte are known as capacitation. It lasts between 5 and 15 hours and takes place in contact with the uterine fluid and in the oviducts, inducing surface changes that enable the spermatozoa to adhere to the egg's vitelline membrane. Only 1% of the initial spermatozoa survive and undergo capacitation. Then only around twenty per oocyte quickly reach the ampulla, usually 1 hour 30 to 2 hours after oocyte emission. Penetration by a spermatozoon causes the zona pellucida to harden, so polysperm penetration is not possible.

IV.3. Descent of the ovum and fertilisation :

Transport of the ovum into the ampulla takes place in a few minutes and is dependent on muscular contractions and ciliary beats which are themselves controlled by restradiol sëcrëtë from the ruptured follicles. Fertilisation takes place in the oviduct ampulla approximately 12 to 14 hours after coi't. In the absence of oocytes, spermatozoa retain maximum fecundability between 10 and 18 h *p.c.* All embryos are present in the isthmus of the oviduct 24 hours after coitus. The embryos have completed their first cell cycle at 26 h *b.w.*, and then continue to divide to reach the 4-cell (**26-32** h *b.w.*), 8-cell (**32-40** h *b.w.*), 16-cell (**40-47** h b.w.) and 8-cell (40-47 h b.w.) stages.

p.c.), morula (**47-68** h *p.c.*) and blastocyst (**68-76** h *p.c.*) (**Figure 22**).

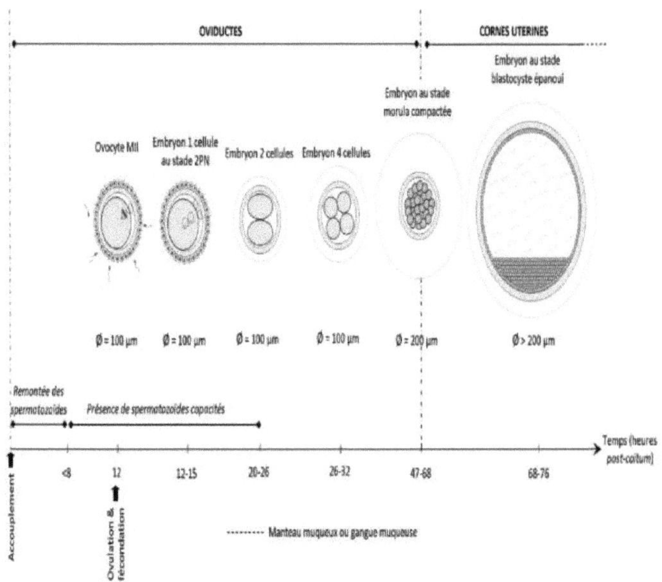

Figure 22: Embryonic development in the rabbit.

The survival of the embryo depends on the two extracellular layers that surround it: the zona pellucida, which is the innermost layer. It is formed during ioliicuiogenesis in the ovaries and the mucous layer, which is the outermost layer. It is put in place during the migration of the embryo into the oviduct, when it increases from 10 pm at 24 hours post-coital in the isthmus to 100 pm at 72 hours post-coital, and plays a vital role in the implantation of the embryo on the uterine wall.

CHAPTER V

V. Gestation :

V.1 Gestation process :

During its passage through the oviduct, the egg divides into blastocysts which reach the uterus after around 4 to 3 and a half days, but the uterine lace will only appear between 5 and 8 days after mating under the action of progesterone. During the 5eme and 6eme days, they develop into a disc-shaped embryonic bud and a trophoblast. At this stage, the blastocyst becomes attached to the uterine mucosa. Initially, a syncytium forms between the cells of the trophoblast and those of the uterus, then the deciduomas rapidly form as the amnion develops. The actual implantation takes place 7 days after mating, at the blastocyst stage.

The developing corpora lutea begin to secrete significant quantities of progesterone, which increase steadily between 3eme and 12eme days after mating, then decrease rapidly in the few days before parturition, while the restrogen secretion undergoes lesser changes. Corpus luteum is essential and remains until the end of gestation. The survival of corpora lutea in the rabbit is under the control of restrogens sëcrëtësed by the follicles, themselves under the control of FSH and LH, which have a lutëotropic action. From 16-18 days of gestation, the link between the foetal placenta and the dëciduoma is lax enough for sëparation to be easy and therefore all manipulations should be rëalisëes with precaution.

V.2 Embryonic and fretal losses during gestation :

The size of the portae is far from identical to the number of ova laid. This variation is Hëc to embryonic and fretal losses that occur during the various phases of gestation. Approximately 30 to 40% of oocytes released during ovulation die in rabbits. Prenatal survival is a complex parameter that depends on a series of events ranging from gamete maturation to the birth of newborns, namely ovulation, fertilisation, early embryonic division, implantation and embryonic development and then fertilisation.

In the rabbit, three critical periods for survival have been identified. The first is between 8eme and 17eme days of gestation, when the hemochorial placenta completes its development and fretus nutrition begins to be under the control of the placenta. During this period, the fry are not affected by the female's reproductive capacity. The second is observed between 17eme and 24eme days *post cottum*, corresponding to the period of uterine elongation when tension on the spherical conceptus is at its maximum and blood flow to the uterus decreases. Finally, the third period is observed during the last week of gestation when the ënergëtic requirements for fretal growth increase rapidly, while feed intake decreases during the days prior to parturition.

> **The distribution of mortality during gestation :**

- **Losses before implantation :**

Mortality before placentation varies between 10% and 21%. During the preimplantation phase, losses are mainly related to embryo viability (chromosomal abnormalities, oocyte and embryo development), and to the uterine and oviductal environment (the composition of uterine secretions).

- **Losses during placentation :**

During the placentation period, the embryonic losses observed are more related to the characteristics of the embryos themselves than to the conditions of the rabbit's uterine environment. Losses during placentation can reach 2%.

- **Post-placental loss:**

The critical time for fretal survival is between $8®^{me}$ and 17^ days of gestation, when placenta development takes place. In fact, as with other polytoid species, the prenatal losses observed during this period seem to be linked to the development of the placentas, itself influenced by the availability of space (**Figure 23**) or the uterine capacity of the female and by the vascularisation of the uterus in the rabbit. The

Overcrowding of the uterine horn in rabbits results in the embryos being crowded together, causing competition between them and between their placentas for uterine space and, consequently, a reduction in fetal survival. The percentage of mortality is generally low and varies according to the authors. In general, there are two peaks in mortality after implantation. Indeed, 66% and 27% of total fetal losses are respectively observed between implantation and the 17eme day of gestation and between the 18eme and the 24eme day of gestation.

The uterine horn

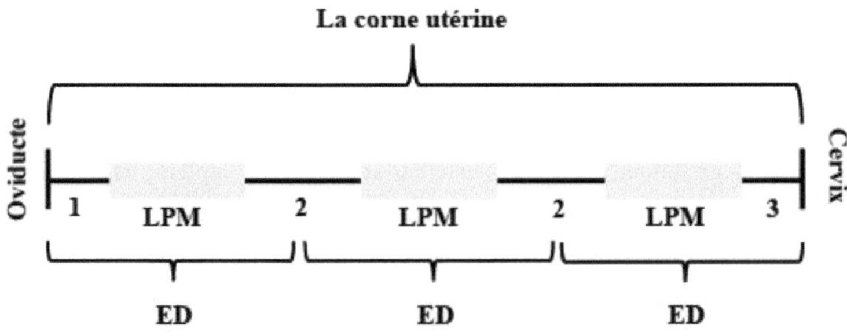

Figure 23: Vital space per fetus measured on the uterine horn.

LPM: Length of the maternal placenta; **ED**: Espace vital or available space for each fetus;
1: Distance between the top of the uterine horn and the first maternal placenta; 2: Distance between two adjacent maternal

26

placentas; **3**: Distance between the cervix and the first maternal placenta.
placenta.

V.3. Placentation :

In eutherian mammals, the placenta is a transitional organ that ensures metabolic exchanges between the mother and the foetus, protecting it fairly effectively against bacteria and toxic substances. It also has an endocrine activity that is responsible in whole or in part for the hormonal balance of gestation. In the rabbit, a placenta is formed at each junction between the fetus and the uterine wall, with the maternal part developing first and reaching its maximum weight at around 16eme days gestation. The foetal part is visible from around 10eme days, and its weight exceeds that of the maternal placenta from 21eme days of gestation (**Figure 24**).

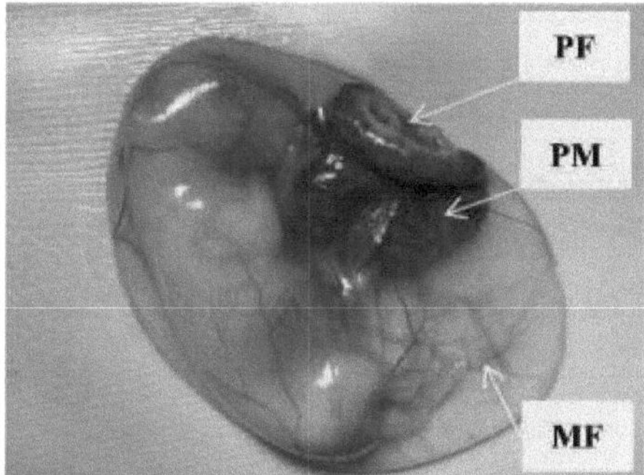

Figure 24: Fretus, fretal membranes and placentas. PF: fetal placenta; PM: maternal placenta; MF: fretal membranes.

- Characteristics of the placenta in rabbits :
The placenta in rabbits differs from that of other domestic mammals in the following ways (**Table 2**):

> **Deciduous placenta (or deciduous placenta)**: the maternal-freetal interdigitations are deep and branched, resulting in haemorrhage associated with tissue loss at the time of delivery.

> **Hemochorial placenta**: the trophectodermal epithelium is in direct contact with the maternal blood at the level of the blood lakes. Maternal-foetal exchanges are easier, with food nutrients passing through only three layers: the epithelium, the connective tissue and the foetal endothelium.

> **Discoid placenta**: appears as a discoid mass.

Table 2: Classification of placentas from different species.

Classification according to endometrial damage		
	Indecidue	**Decidue**
Ruminants	+	
Carnivores		+
Rabbit		+
Mare	+	

Classification according to morphological variations				
	Broadcast	**Cotyledonaire**	**Zonaire**	**Discoide**
Ruminants		+		
Carnivores			+	
Rabbit				+
Mare	+			

Classification according to structural variations				
	Hemochorial	**Endotheliochorial**	**Syndesmochorial**	**Epitheliochorial**
Ruminants			+ (Goat, ewe)	+ (Cow)
Carnivores		+		
Rabbit	+			
Mare				+

V.4. Diagnosis of pregnancy :

In order to rationalise breeding, it is necessary to diagnose pregnancy as quickly as possible. The pregnancy test, which consists of periodically putting the female in the male's cage and waiting for his reaction, is not reliable. In fact, some females accept mating when they are full, others refuse it when they are not. Generally speaking, a pregnant female rabbit becomes aggressive and her re-presentation to a male is always followed by a fight. To avoid the risk of abortion, other diagnostic methods are used.

> **Diagnosis of pregnancy by abdominal palpation :**

Pregnancy checks are carried out between the tenth and fifteenth day after mating. At this stage, the embryos are sufficiently developed to be detected through the abdominal wall.

- Technique:

To do this, one hand grasps the skin above the kidneys and lifts the hindquarters, the other hand passes gently under the abdomen at the level of the belly and, with a back and forth movement, the embryos are located in the form of small soft balls that are slippery to the touch in the event of gestation (**Figure 25**). Palpation before day 10®^me is ineffective, and after day 15®^{me} there is a risk of abortion.

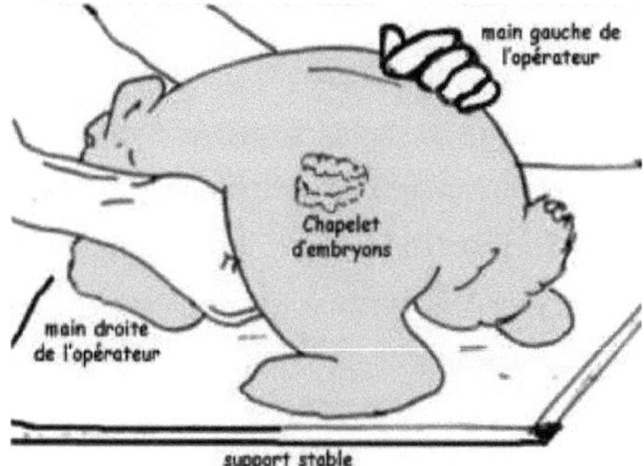

Figure 25: Diagnosis of pregnancy by abdominal palpation.

> **Diagnosis of pregnancy by ultrasound :**

In lagomorphs, ultrasonography of the genital tract is the indication of choice. In addition to determining the presence or absence of pregnancy, it is possible to monitor foetal development accurately. This technique can also provide evidence of certain pathologies of the reproductive system (тёйс, pyomëtre). It is possible to make a diagnosis of gestation by ëchography as early as 7®^{me} days of gestation through the visualisation of embryonic vësicles (**Figure 26**). These vësicles are approximately 8 mm in size and can be counted from day 8®^{me} . They gradually increase in size to reach 17mm around 10®^{me} day.

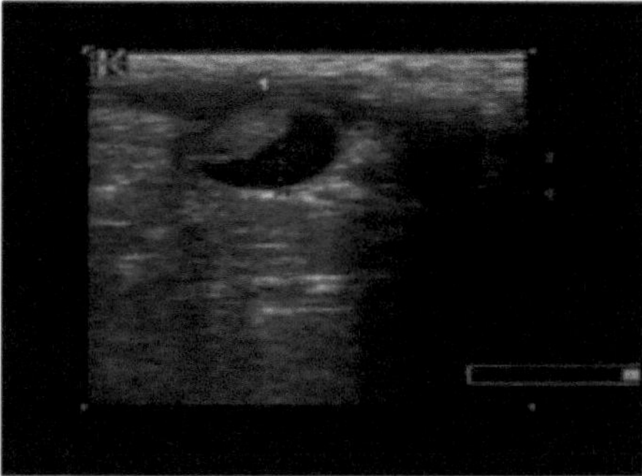

Figure 26: The embryonic vësicle on day 9®^{me} of gestation in rabbits.

V.5. Pseudogestation :

The ova laid may fail to develop, either due to a lack of fëcondensation (overlap between females or any other stimulation of ovulation without depletion of semen), or due to fëcondensation deficiency (male too young, sterile but sexually active or vasectomised male, insufficient semen quality or even early embryonic death). Despite this, De Graaf follicles are transformed within a few hours into progestational corpora lutea which remain active for 15 to 19 days, preventing any further ovulatory egg-laying. This is the phënomëne of pseudogestation, also known as nervous pregnancy. Initially, the corpora lutea develop and the uterus evolves in the same way as during gestation, but they do not reach the size or progesterone production levels of gestational corpora lutea. Progesterone levels increase during the first 12 days and then start to decline, disappearing between day 15®[me] and day 18®[me] (**Figure 27**). The end of pseudogestation is accompanied by the appearance of maternal behaviour and nest building associated with the rapid fall in progesterone levels.

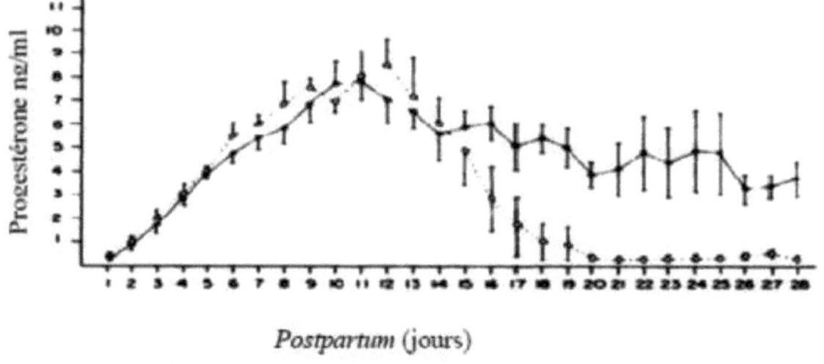

Figure 27: The sëric concentration of progërone in pregnant - and pseudogestating 0 rabbits.

VI. Giving birth :

Parturition is the set of mechanical and physiological phases that lead to the expulsion of the foetus and its appendages from the female genital tract at term. All these phenomena are under endocrine control as a result of the disruption of the equilibrium established during gestation. In the rabbit, gestation lasts 30 to 32 days, but is sometimes extended to 33 to 34 days. Gënërally, rabbits born after a 32-day gestation period are heavier at birth than those born after a 30-day gestation period.

When the time comes to give birth, the female scratches her litter nervously; this behaviour is observed between 25®^{me} and 27®^{me} days into gestation. At the same time, blood levels of estrogens and progesterone were high (60 pg/ml and 9 ng/ml respectively). Three days before parturition, progestërone levels decrease while restrogen levels increase. The female tries to build a nest using her hair and the rest of her body.

the bedding (straw and shavings) in the most isolated corner; and back away from the nest box (**Figure 28**).

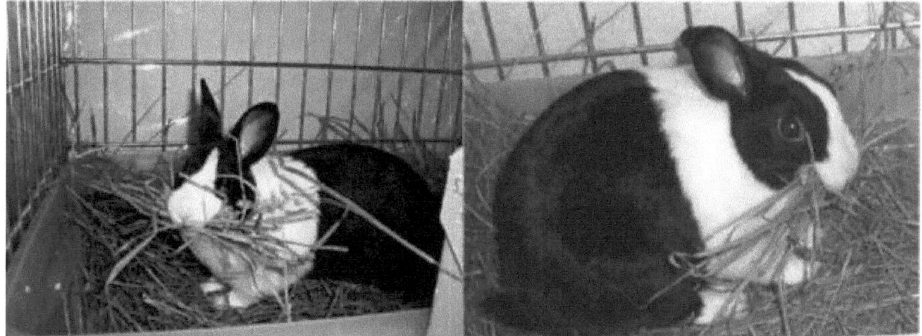

Figure 28: Nest construction.

The hairs used are mainly those on the abdomen; by removing them, the rabbit frees her teats, which facilitates access to the young (**Figure 29**). In addition to its role in keeping the young rabbits at an optimal temperature, the hair has a calming effect via a pheromone called apaisine, which is secreted by the skin of the belly and found in the hair.

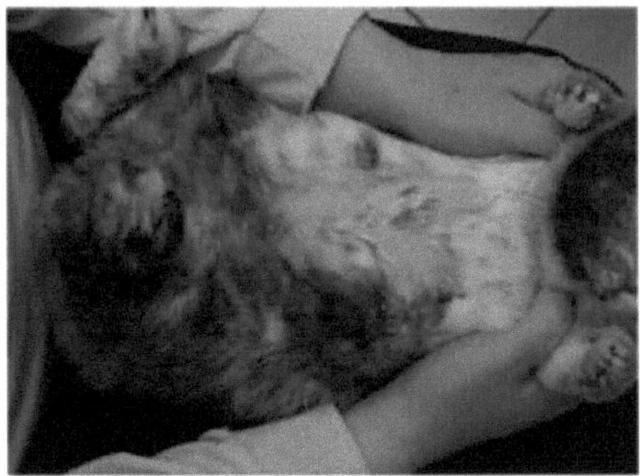

Figure 29: Removal of abdominal hair in a pregnant rabbit.

The mechanism of parturition is relatively poorly understood. It seems that the level of sëcrëtion of corticoids by the surrenal glands of young rabbits plays a role, as it does in other species, in signalling parturition. PGF2a-type prostaglandins also play a role in the initiation of parturition. Corticoids increase placental production of ^strogen, which leads to the onset of lysis of corpora lutea and a reduction in progesterone production. In parallel, a nervous pathway from the distension of the uterus acts on the hypothalamus and completes the impulses from the blood pathway for the production of oxytocin (Ferguson's reflex) (**Figure 30**).

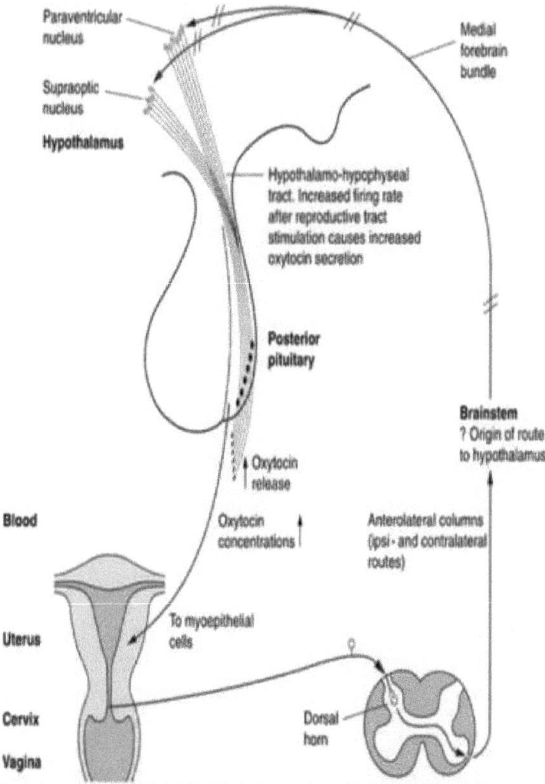

Figure 30: Ferguson's neuroendocrine reflex.

Calving generally takes place early in the morning. It lasts 10 to 14 minutes for large litters and 5 to 7 minutes for medium litters. The female quickly takes care of each youngster as soon as it is born: she cuts the umbilical cord, licks and cleans the residue of freight casings left on their bodies. They then take refuge in the nest and begin to suckle. Rabbits also consume placentas within minutes of giving birth. So the observation of placentas in the nest box more than an hour later can be considered an anomaly.

After giving birth, the uterus regresses very rapidly, losing more than half its weight in less than 48 hours. The rabbit is fertile immediately after giving birth and will be so throughout the lactation period. Regarding the resumption of follicular cycles after parturition, the 1er follicular cycle would begin during the final phase of gestation. As a result, the rate of receptive rabbits (in oestrus) is very high on the day of parturition but decreases rapidly 4 to 5 days later, then rises above 75% around ten days after parturition (**Figure 31**). The 2eme follicular cycle reaches maximum growth on the 9eme *post partum* day.

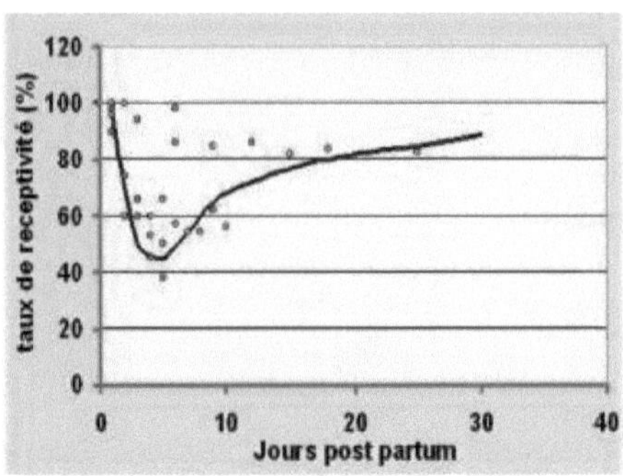

Figure 31: Changes in receptivity during the post-partum period.

VI. Lactation :

At the birth of the young, the mammary gland is perfectly functional but its level of synthesis is still low. At this point, the rapid reduction in progesterone levels and the release of oxytocin stimulate the action of prolactin, allowing the milk to rise. At the time of giving birth, there are 50 to 80g of milk in the rabbit's udder. This type of milk is called colostrum, and its appearance and composition are very different from that of milk (Ig, serum proteins, etc). It is consumed by the young rabbits as they are born.

At each teat, the mechanical stimuli from the rabbits on the teats tend to induce an immediate secretion of oxytocin. Intramammary pressure then increases, allowing milk to be ejected and the young rabbits empty their teats almost completely. A discharge of prolactin (70-75 ng/mL plasma) is observed 1 to 5 min after the end of the tete-a-tete for around 2 to 3 hours, inducing milk synthesis and its accumulation in the mammary glands, at a constant rate, for the next 23 to 24 hours, until the next tete-a-tete.

Rabbits generally suckle their litter only once a day and, although deaf and blind for the first few days, are efficiently guided to the teats (8 to 10 functions) by a pheromone contained in their mother's milk. The young rabbits do not have an attracted teat and change them frequently during the short daily suckling phase (3 to 5 minutes). Lactation in rabbits peaks at around 20-21 days post partum (**Figure 32)** and then increases more or less rapidly depending on their physiological status. It is from the peak of lactation that the young rabbits begin to consume solid feed and go through a transition from milk feed to solid feed, until weaning. Weaning takes place between 28 and 35 days, at a time when the female has practically no milk left.

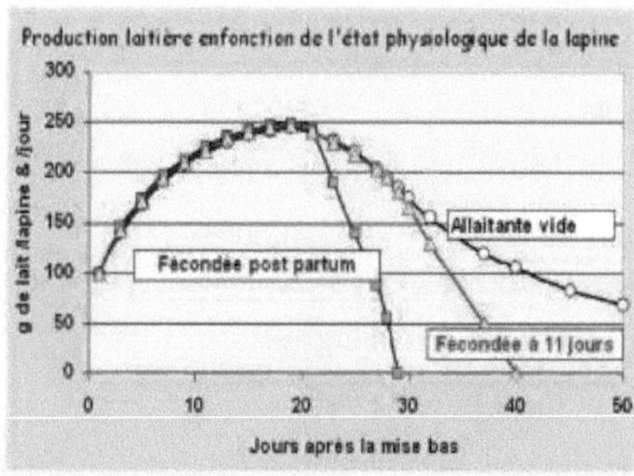

Figure 32: Evolution of production ^Шёгс of rabbits that are simply lactating or simultaneously pregnant and lactating.

Comparative analysis of the milk of some mammifères shows that rabbit milk is significantly richer in protëines, fat and minerals (especially calcium and phosphorus). However, it is very low in lactose (**Table 3**).

Table 3: Comparative composition of cow's, goat's, ewe's and rabbit's milk.

Components in g/kg of milk	Cow	Goat	Ewes	Rabbit
Dry matter	129	114	184	284
Lactose	48	43	44	6
Oils and fats	40	33	73	133
Proteins	33,5	29	58	153
Total minerals (ash)	7,5	8	9	24
Calcium	1,25	1,30	1,90	5,60
Phosphorus	0,95	0,90	1,50	3,38
Magnesium	0,12	0,12	0,16	0,37
Potassium	1,50	2,00	1,25	2,00
Sodium	0,50	0,40	0,45	1,02

VII.Reproductive rhythms :

The reproduction rhythm is defined by the time interval between two successive births, by setting the minimum time between the birth of a female rabbit and the mating that produces the next litter. This is done in order to control the numerical productivity of the rabbits. The rhythms most commonly used in rabbit farming are :

V   II.1 The intensive or post partum rhythm:

Breeding takes place 1 to 2 days after giving birth. Almost all the female rabbits are in oestrus at this time and accept mating. Mating is carried out with the aim of obtaining maximum productivity, despite a number of disadvantages, such as a reduction in pen size and pregnancy rate.

V   II.2 Semi-intensive rhythm :

Breeding takes place 10 to 12 days after the start. Today, this seems to be the most reasonable and most frequently used rhythm, thanks to the better zootechnical performances obtained.

V   II.3. Extensive rhythm :

Females are bred after weaning. Fertility and receptivity are better, but this rhythm is rarely adopted as it only allows very limited productivity per unit of time and does not use all the rabbit's potential.

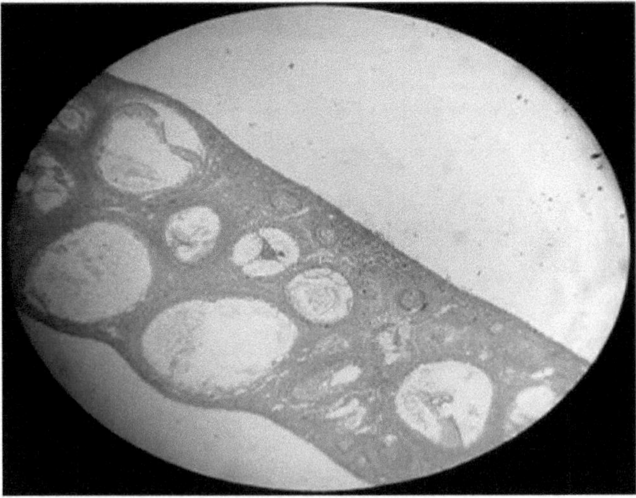

Figure 01: Histological section of the ovary of a **GX40** rabbit (different classes of follicles).

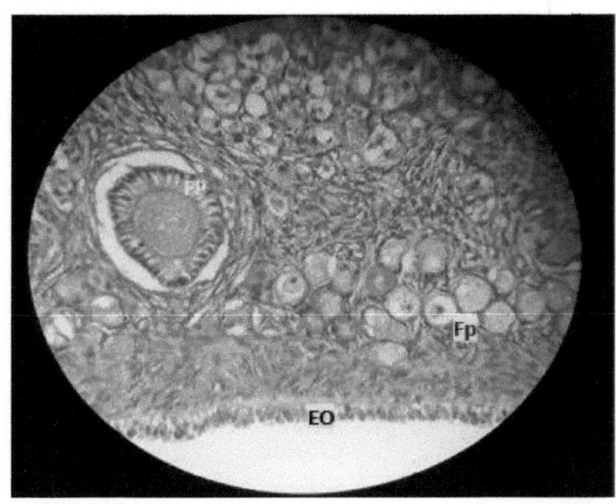

Figure 02: Follicular growth. **Fp**: Primordial follicles; **FP**: Primary follicle; **EO**: ovarian epithelium. **GX100**

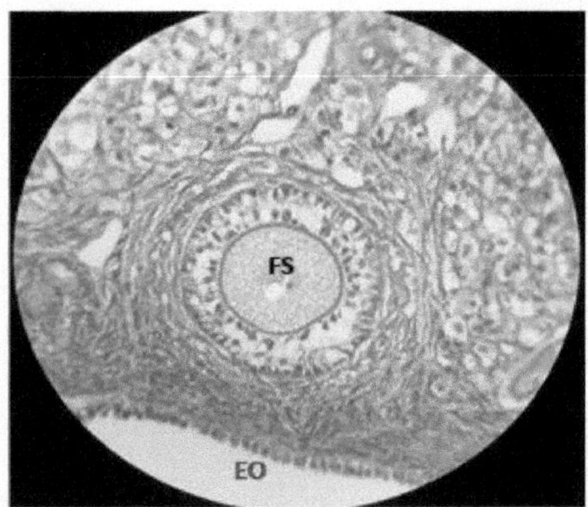

Figure 03: Follicular growth. **FS**: Secondary follicle; **EO**: Ovarian epithelium **(GX10).**

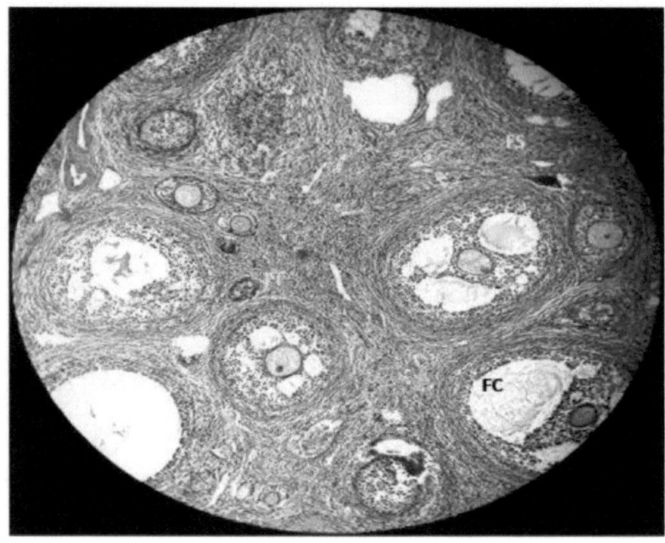

Figure 04: Follicular growth. **FS**: Secondary follicle; **FT**: Tertiary follicle, **FC**: **GX40** cavity follicle.

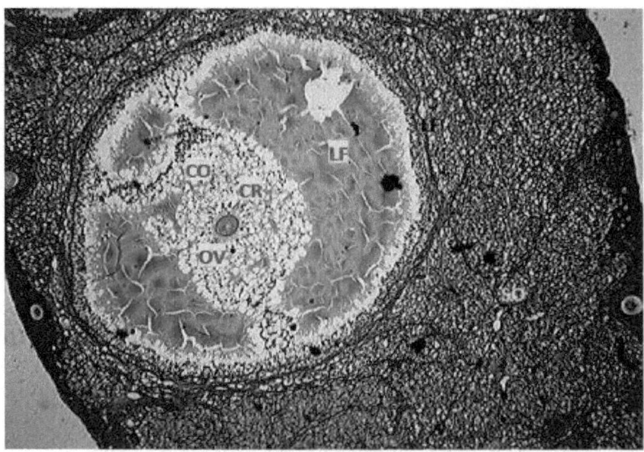

Figure 05: Mature follicle or De Graaf follicle. **OV**: Oocyte; **LF**: Follicular fluid; **CO**: Cumulus oophorus; **CR**: Corona radiata **GX100**.

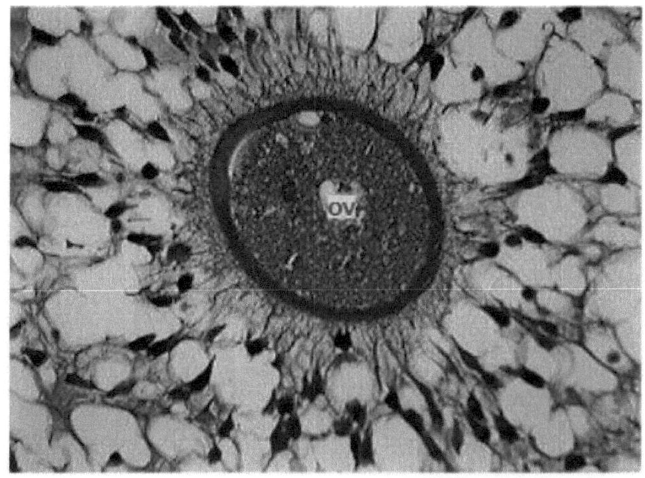

Figure 06: The oocyte of a pre-ovulatory follicle. **OV: GX400** oocyte.

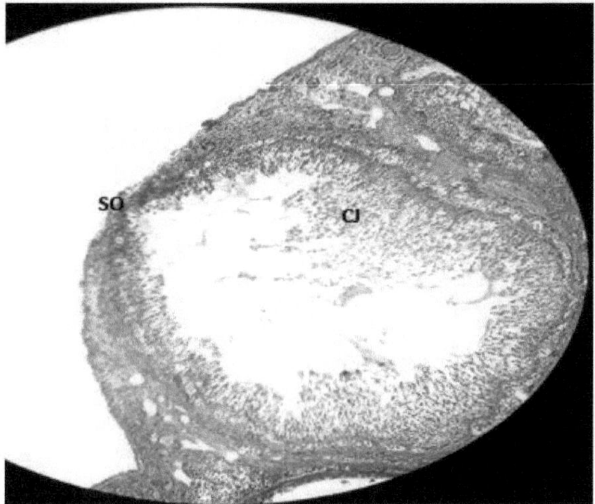

Figure 07: Luteinisation (formation of the corpus luteum). **CJ**: Corpus luteum; **SO: GX100** ovulation stigma.

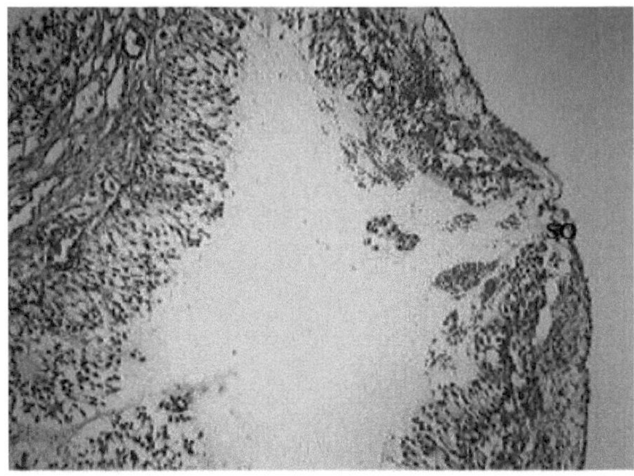

Figure 08: Ovulation (ruptured follicle). **SO**: Ovulation stigma; **GX100**.

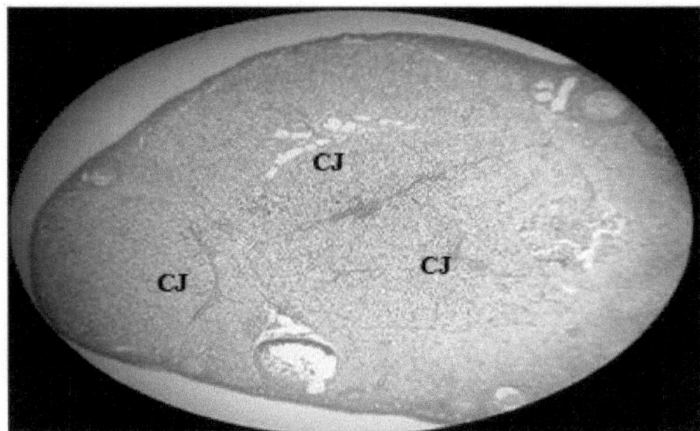

Figure 9: Yellow bodies (**CJ**) **GX100**.

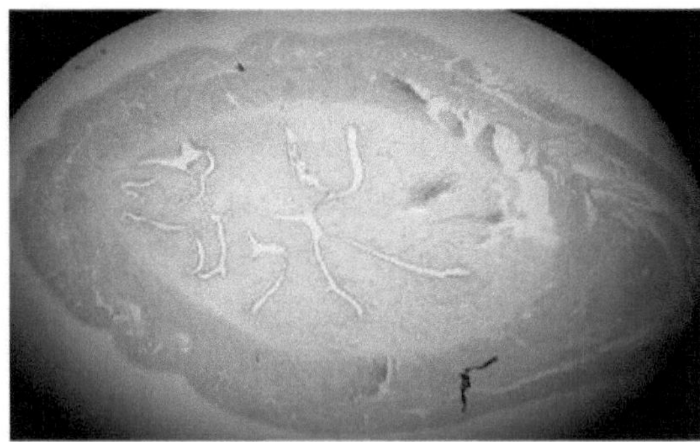

Figure 10: Uterine mucosa in the **GX100** resting phase.

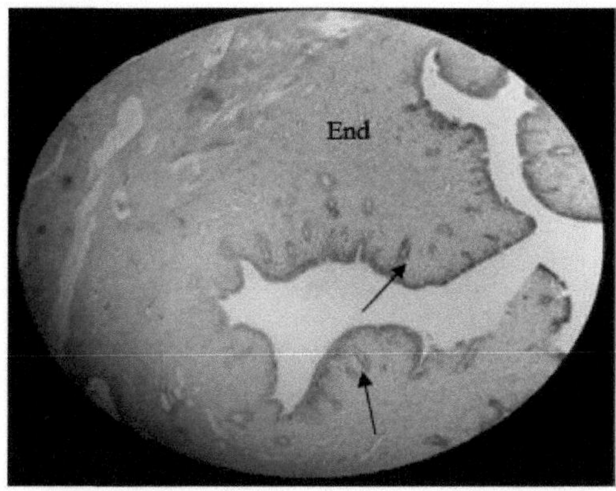

Figure 11: The uterine mucosa: (**End**) Endometrium; **GU:** Uterine glands (arrows) **GX100**.

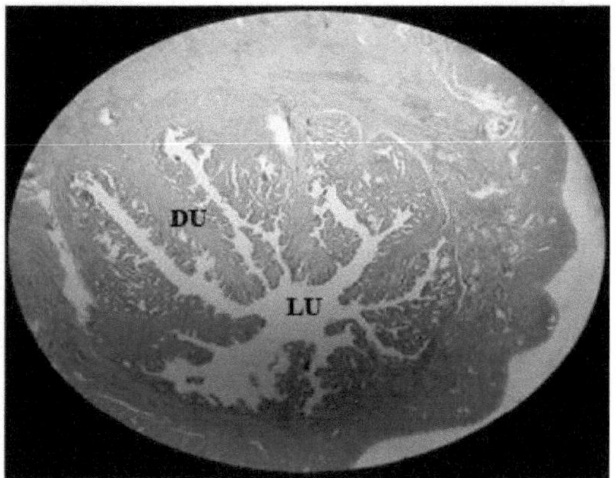

Figure 12: **DU**: Uterine lace formation; **LU** : Uterine lumen in the **GX100** growth.

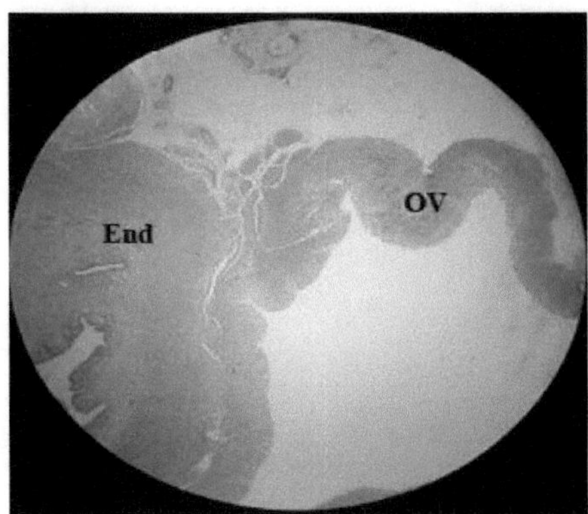

Figure 13: Histological section through the uterus and oviduct. **End**: Endometrium; **OV** : Oviducte **GX100**.

References

Adams G.P., Ratto M.H., Huanca W., and Singh J., 2005. Ovulation-inducing factor in the seminal plasma of alpacas and llamas. *Biology of Reproduction*, 73, 452-457.

AFC and ITAVI, 1998. Memento de l'éleveur des lapins, питёго hors-serie de la revue " *Cuniculture* " Mars/Avril 1988, 7eme edition.

Argente M.J., Santacreu M.A., Climent A., and Blasco A., 2008. Effect of intra uterine crowding on available uterine space per fetus in rabbits. *Livestock Science*, 114, 211219.

Barone R., 1973. Atlas d'anatomie du lapin. 2eme edition. Masson, 91-95.

Belabbas R., 2009. Etude des principales composantes biologiques de la prolificite et facteurs de variation du poids icetnl chez la lapine de population locale (*Oryctolagus cuniculus*). *Magistere en Sciences Veterinaires, Option : Elevage et Pathologie Avicole et Cunicole*, Ecole Nationale Superieure Veterinaire, Alger, 141p.

Belabbas R., 2017. Caracterisation des performances de reproduction ciez le lapin de population locale. *These de doctorat Es-sciences, Specialite : Sciences Veterinaires*, Universite Saad Daileb, Blida I, 258p.

Bencheikh N., 1995. Effet de la frequence de collecte de la semence sur les caracteristiques du sperme et des spermatozoi'des recoltes chez le lapin. *Annales de Zootechnie*, 44, 263 -279.

Berepubo N.A., Nodu M.B., Monsi A., and Amadi E.N., 1993. Reproductive response of pre pubertal female rabbit to photoperiod and/or male presence. *World Rabbit Science*, 1(2), 83-87.

Bodnar K., Torok I., Hejel P., and Bodnar E., 1996. Preliminary study on the effect of ejaculation frequency on some charactertics of rabbit semen. *6th World Rabbit Congress*, Toulouse, 41-44.

Bolet G., Garcia-Ximenez F., and Vicente J.S., 1992. Criteria and methodology used to characterize reproductive abilities of pure and crossbred rabbits in comparative studies. *Option Mediterraneennes, seminar series*, N°17, 95-104.

Bonnes G., Desclaude J., Drogoul C., Gadoud R., Jussiau R., Le Loc'h A., Montmeas L., and Gisele R., 2005. Reproduction des animaux d'élevage. 2eme edition, Edition: Educagri, 407p.

Boumahdi Z., Belabbas R., Theau-Clement M., Bolet G., Brown P., and Kaidi R., 2009. Behavior at birth and anatomo-histological changes studies of uteri and ovaries in the *postpartum* phase in rabbits. *European Journal of Scientific Research*, Vol 34, N° 4, 474-484.

Bourdage R.J., and Halbert S.A., 1988. Distribution of embryos and 500-microM microspheres in the rabbit oviduct: controls for acute motion analysis during transport. *Biology of Reproduction*, 38, 282-291.

Boussit D., 1989. Reproduction and artificial insemination in rabbit farming. Edition Association Frangaise de cuniculture, 233p.

Bouvier A.C., and Jacquinet C., 2008. Pheromone in rabbit: Preliminary technical results on farm use in France. *9th World Rabbit Congress*, Verona, Italy, June 10-13, 303-308.

Bunaciu P., Cimpeanu I., and Bunaciu M., 1996. Mating frequency effect on spermatogenesis and performance of breeding rabbits. *6th World Rabbi Congress*, Toulouse, 51-54.

Chavatte-Palmer P., Laigre P., Simonoff E., Challah M., Chesne P., and Renard J.P., 2005. Caracterisation de la croissance in utero par echographie chez la lapine. *ii^{emes} Journees de la Recherche Cunicole*, 29-30 novembre 2005, Paris, 83-86.

Chretien F.C., 1966. A study of the origin, migration and multiplication of the germ-cells of the rabbit embryo. *Journal of Embryology Experimental Morphology*, 16, 591-607.

Driancourt M.A., 2001. Regulation of ovarian follicular dynamics in farm animals. Implications for manipulation of reproduction. *Theriogenology* 55, 1211-1239.

Fayez M., and Rashwan A., 2003. Rabbits behaviour under modern commercial production conditions. *Arch. Tierz, Dummerstorf,* 4, 357-376.

Foote R.H., and Carney E.W., 2000. The rabbit as a model for reproductive and developmental toxicity studies. *Reproductive Toxicology*, 14, 477-493.

Gabery, 1992. Les lapins : races-soins-elevage. Published by Rustica. Paris.

Gallouin F., 1981. Physiological mechanisms of reproduction. Etat endocrinien de la lapine apres l'ovulation. *Cuniculture*, 8 (6), 294-297.

Gayrard V., 2007. Physiology of mammalian reproduction. Ecole Nationale Veterinaire Toulouse, September, 198p.

Giannetti R., 1984. L^levage rentable du lapin. Publisher: Vecchi, 191p.

Gonzalez M.J., 2004. Maternal behavior in rabbit: regulation by hormonal and sensory factors. *8th World Rabbit Congress*, Puebla (Mexico), September, 1218-1228.

Hawk H.W., 1982. Effect of acetylcholine, prostaglandins F2a and estradiol on number of sperm in the reproductive tract of inseminated rabbit. *Journal of Animal Science*, 55(4), 891-900.

Hill M., 1933. The growth and regression of follicles in the oestrous rabbit. *Journal of Physiology*, 80, 174-178.

Hulot F., and Mariana J.C., 1985. Effect of gënotype, age and season on preovulatory follicles of the rabbit 8 hours after mating. Reproduction Nutrition and Development, 25, 17-32.

Iles I., Boukhari S., Belabbes R., Boulbina I., Zenia S., and AinBaaziz H., 2013.

Relationship between external characteristics of the vulva and sexual behaviour in the domestic Aigerian rabbit. *Livestock Research for Rural Development*, 25, (8), 2013.

Joan Y., Landis Keyes P., and Richard C., 1980. Comparison of serum Progesterone, 20 a-Dihydroprogesterone and Estradiol-17e in pregnant and pseudopregnant rabbits: evidence for posimplantation recognition of pregnancy. *Biology of reproduction*, 23, 1014-1019.

Johnson M.H., and Barry J., 2002. Reproduction. *Sciences Medicales serie Pasteur.* Edition: DE BOEK universite, 298p.

Kranzfelder D., Korr H., Mestwerdt W., and Maurer-Schultze B., 1984. Follicle growth in the ovary of the rabbit after ovulation-inducing application of human chorionic gonadotropin. *Cell Tissue Research*, 238, 611-620.

Lebas F., Coudert P., De Rochambeau H. and Thebault R., 1996. Rabbit breeding and pathology. FAO. Edition : Rome, 227p.

Lebas F., 2018. Cuniculture, rabbit biology. www.cuniculture.info (accessed 10/04/2018).

Machet E., 2006. Caracterisation de la croissance icetale in utero par echographie chez la lapine. *These pour le Doctorat Veterinaire*, la Faculte de Medecine de Creteil, France, 89p.

Mariana J.C., and Solari A., 1993. Proliferation of follicular cells and the effect of FSH on the onset of follicular growth in the ovary of 30-day old rabbits studied by continuous labelling with 3H-thymidine. *Reproduction Nutrition Development*, 33, 63-67.

Marongiu M.L., and Gulinati A., 2008. Ultra sound evaluation of ovarian follicular dynamics during early pseudopregnancy as a tool to inquire into the High progesterone syndrome of rabbit does. *9th World Rabbit Congress*. Verona, Italy, June 10-13, 393398.

Millis T., Copland A., and Osteen K., 1981. Factors affecting the post ovulatory surge of FSH in the rabbit. *Biology of reproduction*, 25, 330-335.

Nizza A., Di Meo C., Taranto S., and Stanco G., 2001. Effect of collection frequency on rabbit semen production. *World Rabbit Science*, 10 (2), 49-52.

Peters H., Levy E., and Crone M., 1965. Oogenesis in Rabbits. *Journal Experimental Zoology*, 158, 169-179.

Perrot B., 1991. L^levage des lapins. *Collection Verte Armand colin*, 127p.

Prud'hon M., 1975. Le lapin : Regies d^levage et hygiene. Physiologie de la reproduction: Mëthodes de reproduction, 87-106. *Informations techniques des services veterinaires*, N° 51-54.

Quinton and Egron, 2001. Maitrise de la reproduction chez la lapine. *Le point veterinaire*, No. 218, August-September, 28-33.

Quintela L.A., Pena A.I., Barrio M., Viga M.D., Diaz R., Maseda F., and Garcia P., 2001. Reproductive performance of multiparous rabbit lactating does: effect of lithing programs and PMSG use. *Reproduction Nutrition Development*, 41, 247-257.

Ratto M.H., Huanca W., Singh J., and Adams G.P., 2005. Local versus systemic effect of ovulation inducing factor in the seminal plasma of alpacas. *Reproduction Biology Endocrinology*, 3, 29.

Rodriguez J.M., Gosalvez L.F., Diaz P., and Gomez S., 1987. Evolucion de la poblacion de foHculos antrales de la coneja en torno al parto. Inv Agrar: Prod Sanid Anim 2, 65-76.

Salissard M., 2013. La lapine, une espece a ovulation provoquee Mëcanismes et dysfonctionnement associee : la pseudogestation. *These pour obtenir le grade de Docteur Veterinaire,* l'Universite Paul-Sabatier de Toulouse, 105p.

Salvetti P., 2008. Embryo production and oocyte cryopreservation in rabbits: Application to the management of genetic resources. *These de l'Universite de Lyon*, 180p.

Schober J.M., and Pfaff D., 2007. The neurophysiology of sexual arousal. *Best Practice and Research : Clinical Endocrinology and Metaboism*, 21 (3), 445-61.

Smelser G.K., Walton A., and Whetham E.O., 1934. The effect of light on ovarian activity in the rabbit. *Journal Experimental Biology*, 11, 352-363.

Theau-Clement M., 2008. Insemination success factors and methods of oestrus induction. INRA. *Productions Animales*, 21(3), 221-230.

Thibault C., and Levasseur M.C., 2001. La reproduction chez les mammiferes et l'homme. INRA Editions, 928p.

Vicente J.S., Lavara R., Marco Jimenez F., and Viudes-De-Castro M.P., 2008. Rabbit reproductive performance after insemination with buserelin acetate extender. *Livestock Science*, 115, 153-157.

Villena F.E., and Ruiz Matas J., 2003. Livestock Technician, Volume 2, edition Cultural S.A. Poligon industriel Arroyomolinos, 256-266.

Yaou A., Kpodekon M., and Lebas F., 2009. Mëthodes et techniques d^levage du lapin : elevage en milieu tropical. www.cuniculture.info (accessed 10/04/2018).

Ypsilantis P., and Saratsis Ph., 1999. Early pregnancy diagnosis in the rabbit by real time ultra sonography. *World Rabbit Science*, 7 (2), 95-99.

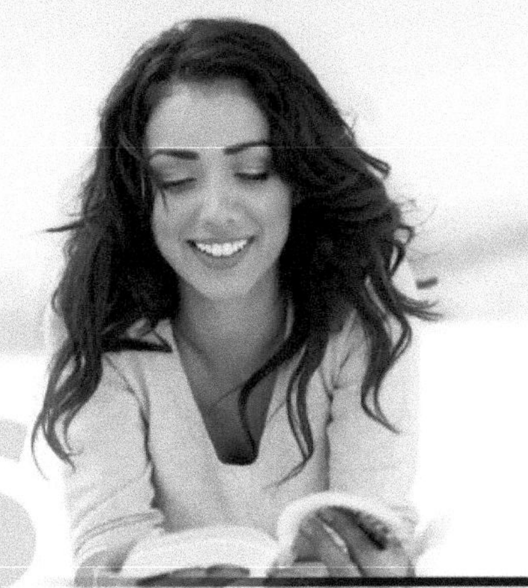

yes I want morebooks!

Buy your books fast and straightforward online - at one of world's fastest growing online book stores! Environmentally sound due to Print-on-Demand technologies.

Buy your books online at
www.morebooks.shop

Kaufen Sie Ihre Bücher schnell und unkompliziert online – auf einer der am schnellsten wachsenden Buchhandelsplattformen weltweit! Dank Print-On-Demand umwelt- und ressourcenschonend produzi ert.

Bücher schneller online kaufen
www.morebooks.shop

info@omniscriptum.com
www.omniscriptum.com

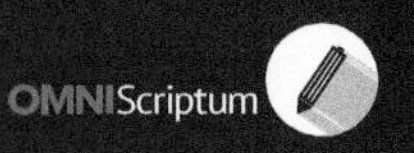

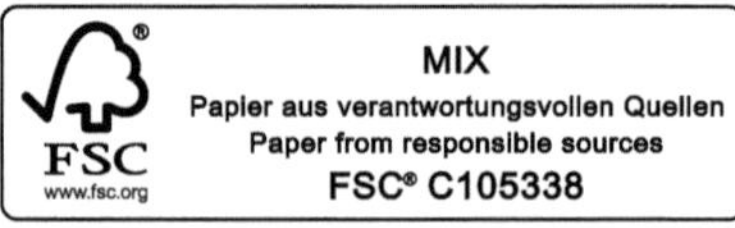

Printed by Books on Demand GmbH, Norderstedt / Germany